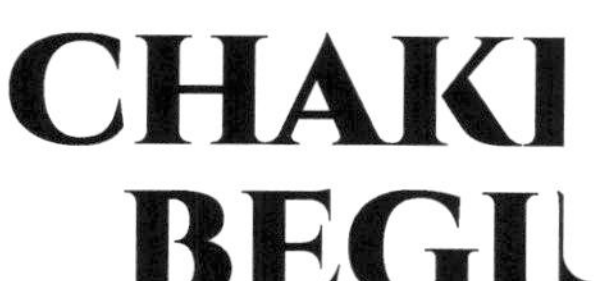

101 Things You Need To Know About Chakras. The Ultimate Beginners Guide to Awaken, Balance and Self Heal Through the Power of Chakras

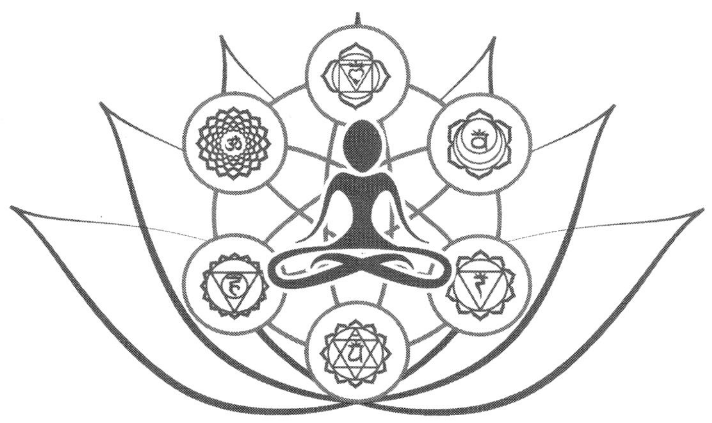

Ella Hughes

The following eBook is reproduced below with the goal of providing information that is as accurate and reliable as possible. Regardless, purchasing this eBook can be seen as consent to the fact that both the publisher and the author of this book are in no way experts on the topics discussed within and that any recommendations or suggestions that are made herein are for entertainment purposes only. Professionals should be consulted as needed prior to undertaking any of the action endorsed herein.

This declaration is deemed fair and valid by both the American Bar Association and the Committee of Publishers Association and is legally binding throughout the United States.

TABLE OF CONTENTS

Introduction

Energy - what does it mean?

To most, energy is power; fuel that keeps our world in motion. From electricity that fires up our homes, to gas that keeps our cars moving, this type of energy is an essential part of our daily life.

To others, *energy* is strength. The capacity to move our bodies, to enact feats that engage our physical capabilities, *to use our bodies* - this type of energy is born from the satisfaction of biological needs. We eat, we rest, and thus, we're recharged with enough energy to see through another day.

Then there are a few others – *us*. People who believe that energy is much more than power for homes or bodily strength. *Energy* is spiritual. It's transcendent and obscure, and if you're willing to understand it and leverage it, you can tap into its extraordinary potential.

Throughout the years, the spiritual concept of *energy* has become more widely accepted and believed, making its way into our households by way of yoga, meditation, and mindfulness. Yet mainstream avenues that share information on this mysterious abstraction fail to truly capture what *transcendent energy means or what it really is.*

Chakras.

Dating back to the earliest religions and spiritual practices known to human civilization, *chakras* are as mysterious as they are powerful. Unfortunately, the concept of these powerful energy centers has been deformed, altered, and modified to fit the ideals of mainstream society. These days, chakras are referenced freely, with most people thinking they fully understand the concepts when they've barely even scratched the surface of their immense and extensive reality.

No doubt, understanding how chakras work, how we can affect them, and what we can do to optimize their flow can be confusing. In particular, if you're only beginning to understand the importance of developing a connection with your energy centers. But if you take the time to discover their origins and learn their intended use, it's possible that you will experience their amazing power at the deepest levels of your spirituality.

So, if you want to learn more about optimizing your chakras and patterning your practices to guarantee a seamless flow of energy - the answer is here.

In this complete guide, you'll learn everything you need to know about chakras, how to work with them, and what you can do maximize their capabilities. This comprehensive book covers *101 essential fragments of knowledge* for chakra beginners, giving you a definitive understanding of all the basics you need to master your chakras.

So now, cosmic warrior, if you're ready to dive in and discover the inherent power that dwells inside your very flesh, read on

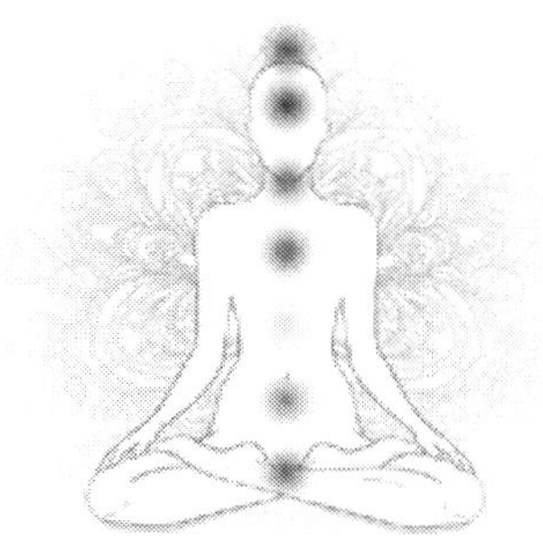

CHAPTER One

A Brief History on Chakras

Since the popularization of yoga as a fitness technique, the word "chakra" has become something of a household term. Unfortunately, the word has also lost quite a bit of its original meaning, since many yoga instructors and enthusiasts fail to truly understand where the concept comes from.

This lack of knowledge on the origins of chakras is the main reason for widespread misinformation on what they exactly are and how they truly work in the body. That's why it's important to firstly develop an understanding of the historical background of these powerful energy centers to properly grasp their truth

1st Thing you need to know…

They Originated In India

The origins of chakras can be traced back to prehistoric India at around 1500 to 500 BC.

Back then, they were documented in an old text called the "Vedas." This ancient collection of information contained some of the oldest scriptures, hymns, liturgical material, and mythological accounts of the Hindu religion.

In Hindu belief, the Vedas were created by Brahma - the first of three gods in the Hindu trimurti. Brahma inspired rishis with the knowledge and wisdom they needed in order to write the Vedas, and that's how the ancient text came to be.

The original Vedas revealed information about "cakravartin", which directly translates in to the word wheel. They are referred to as wheels due to their association with a vortex of spinning energy.

2nd Thing you need to know...

There are More Than Just 7

Believe it or not, there are actually ***88,000 chakras*** distributed throughout your body. These energy centers are present over every inch of your skin and inside your system. In some practices, it's said that these chakras are interconnected.

For instance, reflexology – a popular alternative medicine - claims that manipulation of various points on the palms and soles of the feet can relieve ailments throughout other parts of the body. These "pressure points" are said to be energy centers where small collections of spiritual energy are concentrated.

Since they were first discovered however, 7 of the 88,000 chakras were given primary importance. These 7 chakras - aligned along the area of the spine were said to be the most powerful concentrations of energy throughout the body. Tapping into these centers would produce the most pronounced effects on the system, making them of utmost importance to Hindu believers and yogis.

3rd Thing you need to know...

They Tie In Closely With Yoga

One of the reasons why chakras have become particularly well-known today is because of the popularization of yoga as a fitness routine. Unbeknownst to modern yoga practitioners though, the original use of yoga was far less for flexibility and physical fitness.

The origins of yoga are fairly unclear since the practice was passed down through oral storytelling. Some of the earliest information on yoga was transcribed on leaves which were destroyed and lost just a few years after they were written.

What we do know, however, is that yoga dates back over 5,000 years. According to some scholars, the practice was used by early Hindu believers as a way of tying their physical self to their spiritual facet.

The information shared in the ancient Vedas gave them an understanding of their gods as well as their power over the lives of believers. Practicing yoga helped attune their physical bodies with their spirit through energy management, and made it possible for them to "reach" the gods.

The history of chakras is extensive; however, these three facts are the perfect introduction to help guide you towards the correct management of these intricate energy centers.

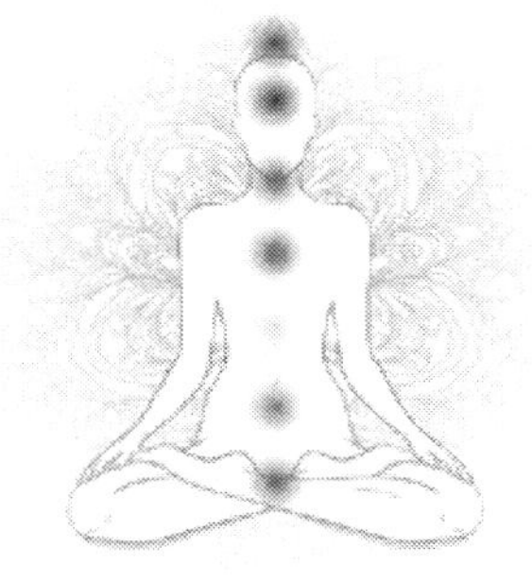

CHAPTER

Two

Common Misconceptions About Chakras

As a beginner in the practice of channeling your chakras, it's likely that you've tried to scour the web for information on how you can make the most of your new practice.

But be cautious - the internet can be riddled with inaccuracies, leaving budding chakra students like yourself with poorly formulated concepts that don't do justice to the original practice and don't maximize the effort you put into channeling your energy centers.

4th Thing you need to know...

Performing Yoga Doesn't Guarantee Chakra Healing

At the end of a yoga class, you may have heard your instructor ask whether you felt relief, or if you feel that your chakras have been cleansed, balanced or open. Maybe if you've been attending classes for years - and I'm talking decades – then this becomes a possibility. But simply completing a few sessions of your monthly yoga classes definitely won't result to healing or clarity.

The earliest Hindus were believed to have spent their whole lives trying to tap into their chakra centers by shifting their entire consciousness and spirituality to tap into these delicate plexuses of energy, so it definitely isn't a process which can happen overnight as you may have been led to believe.

With that being said however, yoga is an amazing practice which helps maintain your fitness levels and helps aid your overall health and peace within, which is important for balancing your chakras.

5th *Thing you need to know...*

Not All Chakra Healers Can Balance Your Chakras

We've all seen them before - alleged experts in chakra healing who can help you balance your energies with different methods that tap into your chakras. While we'd all love to experience the benefits of cleansed energy centers, you need to understand that in our modern age, spiritual healing has become a *big business.*

Lots of clients pay hundreds of thousands to have their chakras cleansed and balanced, and claim that the feeling of relief and clarity can overcome them in as easy as a session or two. Unfortunately, that sense of peace is more often the result of the power of suggestion rather than the effects of the healing session on your chakras.

Keep in mind that for chakra healing to occur, you need a whole consciousness transformation. This means you need to actively seek clarity and cleansing, and you need to be a dynamic part of the change. Simply sitting down and accepting the healing would rarely take effect, more so if you're not visiting the right healer or if you're hoping to achieve instant relief.

That's not to say however that all healers are incapable. Some people are especially gifted when it comes to their capacity to manipulate chakras. If you're careful enough to do your research, you might find one of these talented healers.

6th Thing you need to know...

Chakras Aren't Fixed Temporal Centers

When we look up chakras on the internet, it's possible that you might have encountered diagrams and sketches depicting how they look, the colors they possess, and where precisely they're located on our bodies. While it isn't wrong to assume that the chakras have specific places in our system, it's equally necessary to understand that chakras are not fixed physical centers that we can examine like our organs.

They change, move, and they're definitely not perceivable with the 5 human senses. To fully understand their nature, we must accept that they do not follow the laws of physics and science the way that we've been taught. They operate independently of the tangible world because they're found on a completely different plane all together.

7th Thing you need to know…

An Open Chakra Is the Best Chakra

This is something which we hear about often. The truth is, an open chakra isn't always a good idea for everyone. What most people are looking for and should aim for with chakra healing is to have balanced chakras.

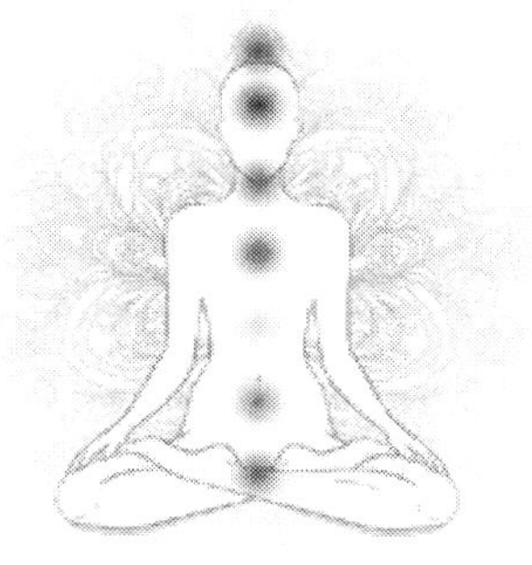

CHAPTER

Three

Basic Chakra Truths

So maybe your concept of chakras was a little shaken up by what you read in the previous chapter. And you might be asking yourself, what should I believe now? What's fact and what's fiction? How do you know whether the things you've learned about chakras are actually truthful or not?

The knowledge of chakras is deep, extensive, and confusing all on its own. Nonetheless, here are some of the basic chakra realities that you can trust are 100% reliable.

8th Thing you need to know...

Combinations of Healing Can Work

In the previous chapter, it was mentioned that pranic healing as well as yoga can't exclusively open or heal your chakras. Certain object associations also have very little proof to them, and may or may not work when it comes to tapping into your energy centers.

What you can believe however, is that chakra healing can occur if you use a combination of these techniques. There is no single method that has been proven to be more effective than other and each of these choices have people who believe in them and people that don't. What's important is that you are proactively using them to improve your current state.

Remember that chakra healing is an experience for your whole being. It takes an active effort to learn, improve, and change your consciousness. The way that happens is through meditation, yoga, and whatever ancillary practices - like crystal healing - you might choose.

No matter the methods you leverage, the possibility of healing depends on your own willingness to be healed. If you believe in what you're doing, you're more likely to experience benefits.

All I would advise you to do is manage your expectations. It could take a lifetime before your efforts produce truly significant changes in your spiritual energy, but if you're dedicated to the methods you choose and you trust in their effects, you will experience their benefits.

9th Thing you need to know...

Healing Takes Place 24/7

There is no rule as to what time of day you should practice your yoga, meditation, mindfulness, or any other chakra healing method you've chosen. But that doesn't mean that the time you spend performing these overt healing techniques is the only time you should focus on healing.

Healing your chakras involves constant, daily effort. It happens while you eat, work, study, or play - it happens throughout your waking hours. It's fueled by consciousness and your deliberate effort to make sure that everything you do throughout the day is performed in the best interest of your chakras.

So, you can't expect healing after a yoga

session if you're going to spend the rest of your day nitpicking your ex-best friend's Facebook profile. You can't anticipate relief after creating a crystal grid if you're allowing stress from work to take over your mental clarity.

You need to be *mindful* of your thoughts, your choices, and your actions. You need to be *fully* invested in making that change. You cannot try to heal your chakras one minute and then indulge in negative or unhealthy behaviors the next.

10th Thing you need to know...

Chakras Can Be Blocked

Many of those who learn about chakras are drawn to one specific truth - they can be blocked. If you weren't originally a believer in the chakra principles, then what might have pushed you to try chakra healing is the knowledge that you might have one that's blocked.

Feelings of anxiety, fear, and tiredness, being unwell, having clouded thoughts - these are just some of the symptoms of a blocked chakra. Maybe you were experiencing similar difficulties in your life without a seeming cause, which is why you turned to chakra healing to find the answer to your discomfort or pain.

Fortunately, you chose the right path. Chakra healing can make you feel healthy, free, and relieved. But because the energy exists on a different plane, you need to be ready to work hard to tap into that deeper level of your being.

11th Thing you need to know...

Chakras Exist On the Subtle Plane

Everything you perceive with your senses can be found on the physical plane. These are things that we interact with daily, and are often the easiest to understand and manipulate. For instance, if you feel an itch on your left elbow, you'll know precisely what it will take to relieve the annoying sensation. If you have a runny nose, then you know you might be coming down with something.

We interact with the physical plane heavily, so most of our actions, thoughts, and feeling are molded to coincide with what we perceive. Unfortunately, this dense physical plane is also what makes it hard for us to tap into the other planes of existence.

The chakras exist on the ***subtle plane*** - or subtle body. This layer of existence is said to reside between the physical and the causal body - two other bodies that each living creature possesses. According to mystics, the subtle body is what controls the physical body, and consists of the ego, intellect, and the mind.

While it is difficult to encapsulate the meaning and purpose of the subtle body, you can think of it as the gateway to the causal body or the true soul. In satisfying the needs of the chakras at the subtle level, you can reach the highest level of clarity, peace, and cleansing of your spirit at the causal level.

12th Thing you need to know...

There Are Major and Minor Chakras

Some resources might say 7, others specify twelve. And then there are some that claim there are over 88,000 different chakras. Yes, it can be overwhelming to think of all the points in your body where energy flows. But you don't have to address every single one of them.

There are primary chakras which are much larger than the rest. It is believed that while each chakra - even the minor ones - are inherently important - the main chakras can actually enact significant, noticeable change.

They have direct impact on the way our physical bodies feel, which is why these large centers of energy are most commonly given preferential importance.

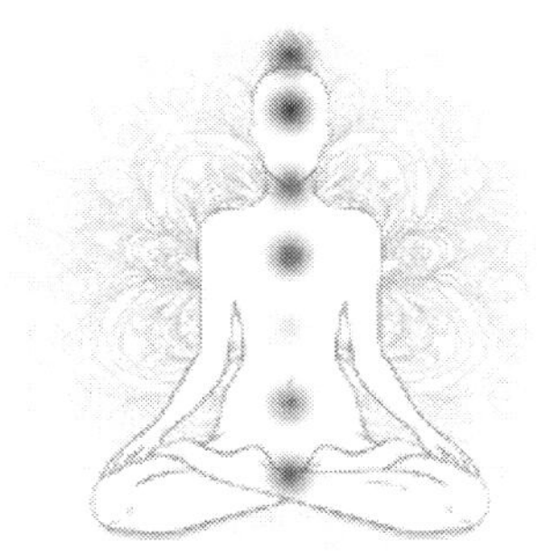

CHAPTER Four

The Main Chakras

Each chakra corresponds to a unique set of ailments, conditions, feelings, and states of being. It's crucial that you address each one with equal preference, so by understanding the nature of individual chakras, it becomes easier to figure out where you need to concentrate your effort to heal.

The number of **primary chakras** changes depending on the reference you've chosen. I'm going to share the 2 most common primary chakra patterns used today.

13th Thing you need to know...

The 7 Chakra System

The most popular chakra system involves just 7 primary chakras. You might have seen them arranged in a line over the area of the spine with one at the top of the head. This chakra system focuses more on you and can be easily correlated to the feelings and symptoms you might experience on the physical body.

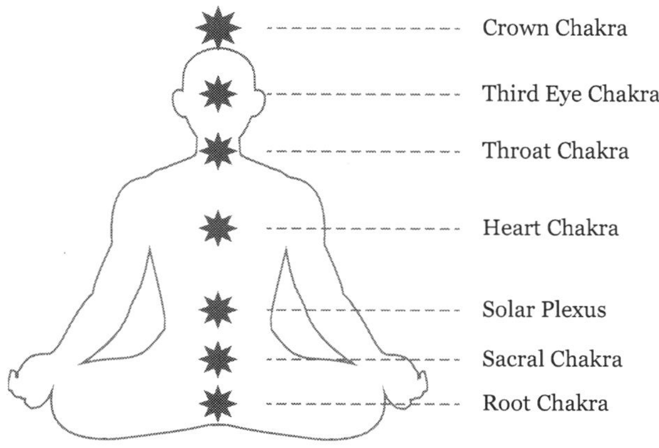

14th Thing you need to know...

The 12 Chakra System

The 12 chakra system on the other hand, provides cosmic warriors with 5 other chakras that aren't found on the body at all. These are the Earth Star Chakra, Soul Star Chakra, Universal Chakra, Galactic Chakra, and Divine Gateway Chakra. The spiritual projections of your soul are found outside of the temporal aspect of your existence, and connect you with the transcendent world around you.

15th Thing you need to know...

Neither Is Wrong

So which system should you subscribe to? First of all, you need to know that neither of these systems is wrong. The 7 chakras are all included in the 12 chakra system, so they basically follow the same standards. The only difference is that the 12 chakra system has 5 other inclusions that you might want to address.

Are these 5 extra chakras as easily manipulated and reached? Not quite, since they're mere projections of your spirit and they don't exist inside your body per se. So, choosing which system you'd like to follow ultimately rests on your preference and your dedication.

16th Thing you need to know...

The Root Chakra

The root chakra is the first chakra in the 12 chakra system and the 7 chakra system. It's also called the "Muladhara" chakra, which is Sanskrit for "foundation."

The purpose of the root chakra is to ground us in our sense of self and our feeling of belonging. It supports the idea of uniqueness and helps in the formation of our identity. So, unlike the earth star chakra (8th chakra) which grounds us to the world around us, the root chakra grounds us in our own self.

17th Thing you need to know...

The Sacral Chakra

Also called the "Svadhisthana" chakra with translates to "one's own abode" or "one's own seat". The sacral chakra is the energy center where we feel pleasure and passion from. This powerhouse encourages thoughts of creativity and joy, and stimulates abundance when properly balanced.

18th Thing you need to know...

The Solar Plexus Chakra

Between the heart and the sacral chakra is the solar plexus chakra. This energy center is where your ego resides, and is responsible for your sense of self as well. The sacral chakra is a storehouse of energy whether it's positive (healing and growth) or negative (fear, pain and stress). A well-balanced solar plexus chakra manifests as assertiveness and willpower, as well as the willingness to act. Its Sanskrit name is "Manipura", with "mani" meaning "gem", and "pura" or "puri" meaning "city."

19th Thing you need to know...

The Heart Chakra

The "Anahata" chakra is the heart chakra, and this Sanskrit name means "unstuck", "unhurt", or "unbeaten." The heart chakras is located in the center of your being and its purpose, as you might have already guessed, is love energy. It's the source of outward love and self love. If your heart chakra is properly balanced, you're likely to experience warmth and compassion.

20th Thing you need to know...

The Throat Chakra

As the fifth chakra in the 7 chakra and the 12 chakra systems, the throat chakra serves the purpose of bridging the lower parts of the subtle body to the upper region. Also called the "Vishuddha" chakra which is Sanskrit for "especially pure," the throat chakra is responsible for your ability to speak, to listen, and to communicate through to higher spiritual beings.

21st Thing you need to know...

The Third Eye Chakra

The third eye chakra, or brow chakra located in the middle of your forehead, is the foundation of your psychic abilities. A third eye chakra that's open or active can give its owner clairvoyance, allowing people to communicate or perceive non-temporal beings in the physical realm. The Sanskrit name for the third eye chakra – "Anja" - means "perceive" or "beyond wisdom."

22nd Thing you need to know...

The Crown Chakra

In the 7 chakra system, the crown chakra or the "Sahasrara" chakra is the last and highest energy center in the body. It corresponds to devotion and a deep sense of the spiritual self. A well-balanced crown chakra can also connect you with higher forces and give you insight on divine forces at work in your life and in the world around you.

The Sanskrit name for the crown chakra means "thousand-petaled" which means that the crown chakra resonates with the most ionic intensity compared to the various other chakras in the 7 chakra system.

23nd Thing you need to know...

The Earth Star Chakra

In the 12 chakra system, the 8th chakra is the earth star chakra. Some label the earth star chakra as the 1st chakra in the 12 chakra system because it's below the root chakra. However, 7 original chakras come before all the extras used in the 12 chakra system
As surprising as it might sound, this chakra is

located a foot and a half below your feet. So, if you were standing upright, it would be one and a half feet in the ground directly below you.

It functions like the root chakra and works to connect you to the core of the earth. It grounds your entire chakra system as well as your etheric body, and may even connect you to your past life.

24th Thing you need to know...

The Soul Star Chakra

While the 7 chakra system ends with the crown chakra, the 12 chakra system carries on with the soul star chakra. This energy center is located just above your head, outside of your physical body. Its purpose is to absorb energy from the world around you and distribute this to the other lower chakras in your body. The Soul Star Chakra is sometimes referred to as the 8th chakra because it comes directly after the crown chakra.

25th Thing you need to know…

The Universal Chakra

Situated above the soul star chakra, the universal chakra connects you to the vast expanse of the universe. Tapping into this chakra and harnessing its power means that you might be able to develop potent psychic as well as powerful healing abilities.

26th Thing you need to know…

The Galactic Chakra

With a well-balanced galactic chakra, you can communicate freely with higher beings. This is why the energy center is also called the "channel for prophecy." Gifted individuals with opened galactic chakras were those who were capable of communicating with beings from other worlds. In many references, it's believed that the original *rishis* were balanced at the level of the galactic chakra, which is why they were able to write the Vedas.

27th Thing you need to know...

The Divine Gateway Chakra

The highest chakra in the 12 chakra system is the divine gateway chakra. Located even higher than the galactic chakra, this energy center exists as a gateway between you and the cosmos. When the divine gateway chakra is properly balanced, you reap the benefits of cosmic freedom. That is, you might be able to freely travel to and from different dimensions with ease.

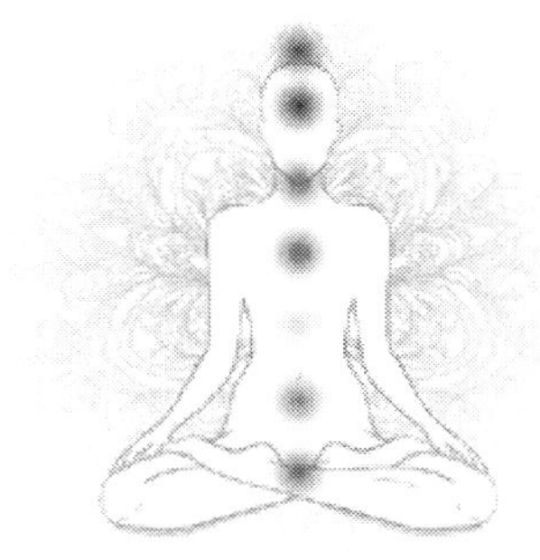

CHAPTER

Five

Associations of the Main Chakras

I mentioned in a previous chapter that any of the associations given to the modern chakra systems as we know them were not actually present in the Vedas. This information sprung when the western world took hold of the chakra concept, starting with Carl Jung who possibly saw similarities between the chakras and the objects and concepts he connected them with.

If you're being strictly traditional about your chakra practice, you might say that the associations lack of Vedic foundation makes them false. But remember that bodies of knowledge change and improve. So, although there hasn't been a lot of research about the reality of the associations, millions of modern day mystics have found that there is some truth to them.

So, what's the importance of knowing these associations?

Understanding the elements, objects, and other factors that chakras are closely linked to can help you detect and localize blockage, and makes it possible to address problems with energy flow more accurately.

28th Thing you need to know...

Each Chakra Has A Color Counterpart

Corresponding colors help add a visual aspect to the chakras. For cosmic warriors like yourself, the purpose of the assigned colors is to assist you in imagining the chakras you're trying to tap into. Because humans are sensory creatures by nature, we're most capable of focusing when we have some sort of empirical foundation to think of.

By using the colors that correspond to each plexus, it becomes easier to visualize the energy center you're trying to connect with. This enhances focus and concentration, and helps attune your mind to the goal of your efforts.

Here are the colors that correspond to each chakra on both the 7 and 12 chakra systems:

Chakra (from bottom)	**Color**
Earth Star	Brown, aqua, or seafoam green
Root	Red
Sacral	Orange
Solar Plexus	Yellow
Heart	Green
Throat	Blue
Third Eye	Indigo
Crown	Ultra violet
Soul star	Blue green
Universal	Pearl white
Galactic	Pink orange
Divine gateway	Shimmering gold

29th Thing you need to know...

Chakras Correspond to Organs

There was definitely no mention of any organ associations between the chakras in the original Veda text. But lots of mystics throughout the westernization of the concept believe that these energy centers are closely linked to a variety of internal organs and body parts throughout our system.

If you're experiencing a specific ailment or issue concerning a body part, it's possible to isolate the chakra responsible by checking whether they correspond to that specific organ or part.

Chakra	Organ/Body Part
Root	Spine, rectum, legs, arms, circulatory system
Sacral	Reproductive organs, kidneys, immune system, bowels
Solar Plexus	Central nervous system, liver, pancreas, skin, digestive tract
Heart	Heart, thymus, lower lungs, immune system, circulatory system

Throat	Respiratory system, thyroid, vocal cords, teeth
Third Eye	Eyes, sinuses, pituitary gland
Crown	Pineal gland, nervous system, brain

You'll notice that organ and body part associations only exist with 7 of the 12 chakras. This is because unlike the primary 7, the additional 5 chakras have less to do with the self and more to do with the individual's connection with the world and the universe around them.

That being said, they exist on the subtle plane without overlapping with the physical body. Therefore, they have no corresponding organs or body parts that may manifest with issues or problems.

It's also important to mention that this is the primary reason why some people choose only to focus on the 7 major chakras, instead of including the other 12. Many mystics and cosmic adventurers have used the concept of chakras as a tool for healing. Since the other 5 chakras have no benefit in that respect, many have chosen to do without them in that they don't provide any direct effect on the physical body.

30th Thing you need to know…

They Link To the Elements

Elemental associations were again born from the western influence of chakras. Their use in modern chakra healing is heavily implemented in a lot of the meditation and mindfulness techniques you might have seen other cosmic warriors applying in their practice.

The benefit of harnessing the power of the elements when meditating is that it lets you target specific chakras more precisely. Some chakras are closely associated with one or two elements. So, if that specific chakra is experiencing an energy flow problem, channeling the element linked to it can help make it easier to manipulate its energy.

Element	Chakra
Earth	Root
Water	Sacral
Fire	Solar plexus
Air	Heart
Ether	Throat, third eye, crown

31st Thing you need to know...

Manifestations of Balanced Chakras

A well-balanced, harmonious chakra gives rise to a variety of physical manifestations that you can experience firsthand. This is what most mystics aim for, since the modern practice of tapping into chakras revolves mostly around healing.

When you properly address your chakras and balance the energy that flows through them, you can reap a variety of benefits that tie into your overall health and wellness.

Chakra	When balanced...
Root	Sense of security, prosperity, confidence that basic needs will be met, sense of wellness and strength, digestive regularity, career/work satisfaction
Sacral	Creative freedom, emotional stability, confidence in your capability to adapt to change

Solar plexus	Power over your life and the circumstances you experience, confidence in your decisions, self-assurance, clarity of choices, strong personal opinions and beliefs
Heart	Self-love, compassion for others, strong capacity to empathize with others, ease of forgiveness
Throat	Ease of expression, ability to freely share your truth, connection with the ethereal realm, ease of vocalization
Third eye	Strong intuition, perception of other dimensions and energies, illumination of mystical states, inspiration and creativity
Crown	Trust, devotion, a deeper sense of happiness and contentment, deep connection with the self on a spiritual level

32nd Thing you need to know...

Crystals and Chakras

Crystal healing is one of the most closely linked practices to chakras. It's said that crystals have the least value of entropy since they're near perfect, naturally occurring substances. With the ideal shapes and colors, crystals can vibrate with precision that restores chakras to the ideal resonance.

There are literally thousands of different crystals, and each one is said to serve a unique purpose in healing. However, each chakra does correspond to a specific collection of crystals that they have preferential associations with.

Chakra	Crystals
Root	Red Jasper, Smokey Quartz, Hematite, Garnet
Sacral	Citrine, Carnelian, Orange Calcite, Topaz
Solar Plexus	Tiger's Eye, Citrine, Malachite
Heart	Rose Quartz, Aventurine, Green Jade, Peridot

Throat	Blue Quartz, Sodalite, Aquamarine, Blue Topaz
Third Eye	Lapis Lazuli, Fluorite
Crown	Clear Quartz, Amethyst, Sugilite, Celestine

33rd Thing you need to know...

Chakras Have Symbols

Each chakra comes with a unique symbol that depicts some of its qualities. These symbols have inscriptions and feature several qualities like color combinations and varying numbers of petals.

The petals represent the level of frequency of the energy that flows through its represented chakra. For instance, the root chakra has only 4 petals, while the crown chakra has 1,000.

The inscriptions on the petals are representative of Sanskrit mantras that correspond to each chakra. Repeating these sounds or words as you focus on meditating over a specific chakra is believed to help improve your oneness with that particular energy center.

34th Thing you need to know...

Foods for Each Chakra

Experts claim that food has significant impact on your chakras. Eating the right food for specific energy centers can help relieve blockage and optimize your overall health.

Here are some of the foods associated with each chakra:

Chakra	Food
Root	Carrots, potatoes, onions, garlic, and other root crops, eggs, meat, peanut butter, soy, chives, paprika, cayenne, and pepper
Sacral	Melons, mangoes, passion fruit, coconut, and other sweet fruits, walnuts, honey, almonds, cashews, cinnamon, vanilla, sesame seeds, chia seeds
Solar plexus	Grains, pasta, bread, sunflower seeds, milk, cheese, yogurt, mint, ginger, chamomile, turmeric

Heart	Kale, spinach, green leafy vegetables, green teas, basil, sage, thyme, celery, broccoli, cauliflower
Throat	Lemons, limes, and other citrus fruits, water, herbal teas, fresh fruit juices, apples, pears, plums
Third eye	Wine, grapes, blueberries, raspberries, grape juice, lavender, poppy seeds
Crown	Fasting

35th Thing you need to know...

Signs of Blocked Chakras

When a chakra becomes blocked, it demonstrates unique symptoms that might not manifest with other chakras. In knowing the specific symptoms that tie in with each chakra, it becomes easier to detect where the blockage or imbalance specifically is. (See next page)

Chakra	Symptoms of Blockage
Root	Difficulty feeling safe and secure, worries regarding self-esteem and self-worth, unsatisfied with work or career, inability to sustain basic needs, eating disorders, insecurity
Sacral	Being controlled by your emotions, no sexual desire or too much sexual energy, feeling stuck in a specific negative mood, preoccupation with sexual fantasies
Solar Plexus	Excessive need to control others around you, lack of control, obsession with small unimportant details of daily life, lack of ambition, lots of ideas or plans but no sure strategies on how to execute or achieve them
Heart	Being defensive or guarded, inability to sympathize or empathize with others, depending too heavily on others, jealousy, fear of commitment or intimacy

Throat	Difficulty expressing one's self, challenges listening or understanding others, fear of talking in front of crowds, feeling nervous when talking to others, compulsive lying, constantly trying to rationalize poor choices and bad actions
Third Eye	Inability to see a clear future beyond problems, unrealistic fantasies involving fictional creatures, inability to develop a vision or goal and execute it, mental fogging
Crown	Disconnection with the spirit, disconnection with the body, creating your own imagined world, obsessive interest or attachment to spiritual concepts, closed-mindedness

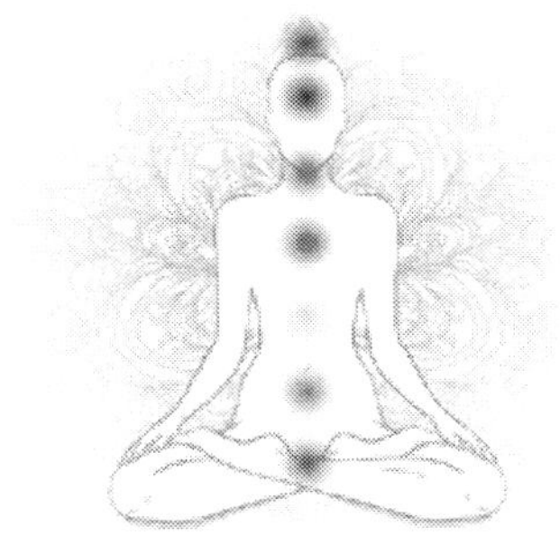

CHAPTER

Six

Healing Your Chakras

The earliest Hindu believers practiced yoga and complete lifestyle adjustments in order to tap into their chakras and balance their energies. They believed that this brought them closer to their gods by becoming the best versions of themselves that they could possibly be.

Today, modern chakra healing focuses on optimizing health and wellness. Many of those who tap into their energy centers are more interested in the therapeutic benefits of the practice, using certain methods to attune to their chakras and address ailments and issues that plague virtually any facet of their being.

Before we dive into the healing practices themselves, it's important to familiarize yourself with the nature of chakras first. This should help make it easier to understand how certain methods might work to improve the flow of energy.

36th Thing you need to know…

They're "Spinning"

When we think of our chakras, we often imagine balls of light, laid out over the length of our spines. While that might not be such a bad way to think of them, lots of scholars and experts believe that our chakras look more like small tornados, spinning steadily as energy flows through and around them.

The funnel-shaped vortexes of light absorb energy from higher bodies and entities, and siphon them down through the lower chakras. All of this energy transfer happens with rhythmical spinning. Each chakra needs to spin at just the right pace to guarantee efficient functionality. If it spins too fast, too slow, or doesn't spin at all, you might experience manifestations of poor chakra balancing.

37th Thing you need to know...

They Can Be Recalibrated

Recalibrating your chakras is the only way that you can balance their energy and experience the benefits of harmony. There are a variety of ways to do this, and most of the modern methods we can leverage are founded on tantric fundamentals.

Essentially, it's ideal that you view your chakras less as transcendent centers and more as an indication of your connection with the world. This makes it easier to manipulate them and tap into them. For instance, someone founded in transcendent belief might find it difficult to reach their chakra because of their sheer distance from the empirical.

However, under tantric fundamentals, it's expressed that the world around us - the empirical realities that we perceive with our 5 senses - is a manifestation of the divine. This way, we can use tools around us specified by western movements in order to tap into our chakras.

Which leads us to the next topic...

38th Thing you need to know...

Methods of Chakra Healing

There is no right or wrong way to heal your chakras, per se. As long as you have the right mentality, it's possible to reach them and optimize their resonance! For instance, one mystic might choose to take a walk through a nature path at least an hour daily in order to balance his energies. Whilst another might choose to sit in silence and meditate. Neither of these methods are wrong - since both are directed towards the same ultimate goal.

That said, deciding on the best healing strategy for yourself depends on what you prefer.

There are a few methods that have been developed throughout the years that are said to be particularly effective at healing blocked or poorly balanced chakras.

39th Thing you need to know...

Crystal Healing

Crystal healing is a practice used around the globe, and is performed by harnessing the energy of crystals. These naturally occurring minerals are said to resonate with the ideal vibrations since they contain the least amount of entropy compared to any other object in the world.

Everything vibrates with energy, so it's believed that the many different realities you encounter daily - from your mobile phone, to the food you eat, to the different items you have in your home - all have an effect on your chakra's vibrations.

Crystal healing aims to restore proper resonance by influencing the movements of your chakras and tuning them to the same pace and frequency. There are a variety of crystals you can use to heal your chakras, and some have special properties for specific uses. A previous chapter discussed the different crystals that target specific energy centers, so please refer to that chart if you decide to try crystal healing.

40th Thing you need to know...

Methods of Crystal Healing

There are a number of different ways that you can leverage crystals to heal your chakra imbalances. Each one requires a different level of effort and skill, but ultimately results to the same outcomes.

Wearing crystals over a specific body part can help target imbalanced chakras. A rose quartz pendant over the chest, for example, can help restore the heart chakra back to proper vibration.

Setting a crystal grid is a more complicated practice and requires quite a higher level of intuition. Crystals are set out in a pattern on a flat surface, and are designed in order to transmit, absorb, and balance energies in a space.

For instance, if you're having issues with feelings of security (a problem associated with the root chakra), setting a crystal grid in your home with earth toned crystals that are used for grounding can help remove negative energies in your space and relieve the disruption in your root chakra.

Swinging a crystal over certain parts of the body can also help restore a problematic chakra.

41st Thing you need to know...

Meditation

Meditation is a thousand-year old practice, calling observers to let go of worldly distractions in order to develop a deeper connection with the self. Meditation isn't as easily performed as mindfulness, but it does provide superior benefits to those seeking relief against chakra disturbances.

Meditation works by requiring mystics to sit in silence and channel their chakras by intense focus. Imagining the chakra spinning and tuning into the flow of energy by pacing your breathing according to the vibrations you sense is a great way to meditate on chakra blockages and imbalances.

42nd Thing you need to know...

Mindfulness

Unlike meditation that requires observers to completely clear their mind and maintain their focus on just one object or chakra, mindfulness is quite the opposite. This method of chakra healing lets you entertain thoughts as they come instead of shutting them out.

In effect, it becomes a lot easier compared to meditation since our physical bodies are prone to having our minds wander and linger on other thoughts. The challenge of mindfulness is localizing the insult to our chakras.

As you engage in a session of mindfulness, your ultimate goal becomes seeking out the issue underlying the symptom you've detected. Which chakra is affected? And how is it responding to the imbalance of energy flow? Allowing your mind to dwell and explore can help shed light on the reality of your chakras' condition.

43rd Thing you need to know...

Massage

How can anything we do at the physical plane have an effect on the chakras located at the subtle plane? Remember that the process of healing relies on tantric foundations.

Therefore, everything we perceive is a reflection

and a direct manifestation of the divine. Our bodies are holy vessels and they're intricately tied into our being. By relaxing the senses, we can get a better perception of our chakras.

Massage is another method of relieving chakra blockages. Those that use specific oils from herbal medicinal plants can be particularly beneficial, especially because certain chakras are closely linked to these plants and natural components.

In Asian cultures, energy called qi could be balanced by way of acupuncture. In many ways, the same belief ties into the way that chakras work, making it a viable option for those who want to relieve chakra imbalances with more relaxing methods that ease the physical plane's distress.

44th Thing you need to do...

Incense

Thanks to western cultures that have brought *tantric* principles to modern day mystics, we now have a variety of methods for chakra healing that were once unknown to ancient yogis and Hindus. For instance, the use of *incense* was widely unknown during the time of the Vedas as a method for tapping into chakras. But today, it's one of the most powerful methods we can leverage.

Engaging the sense of smell helps us tap into latent memories that might have been stored deep within the recesses of our minds. By remembering these suppressed memories, we might be able to discover pains in our being where chakra blockages may have stemmed.

Other than that, science has proven that the use of incense can be very calming. Uses of specific herbs, plants, and extracts that correspond to specific chakras can make the use of incense particularly beneficial towards healing.

45th Thing you need to know...

Affirmations

Remember how it was stated that it doesn't matter how you try to heal your chakras as long as your heart and your mind are in the right place? This *optimized disposition* - the willingness to change for the ultimate good - is what powers the different methods you might use. Whether it's meditation or crystal healing, or everything in between - as long as you *believe* in the right stuff, you're likely to experience relief.

That's what makes the use of *affirmations* so important when attempting to tap into your chakras via any method you might choose. Using these mantras, you can set the tone for your efforts and clear your mind of negativities that might interfere with your journey towards cleansing.

46th Thing you need to know...

Developing an Affirmation

To develop a mantra that's right for you, think about your current situation. What one problem do you want to be released from? It can be something as temporal as your finances to something as abstract as your love life.

Now that you've settled on the issue you want to address, develop a positive mantra that you can repeat to yourself to clear your mind and set your goal. *"I am enough"*, *"I am capable"*, *"I am loved"* are just some examples of mantras you might want to use to help you address an imbalanced chakra.

47th Thing you need to know...

Absorbing Color Vibrations

You'd be surprised to know the kind of power that colors have over our mental well-being and our energy harmony. Of course, it isn't a secret how the human mind associates certain colors with specific feelings and dispositions, which sheds light on their inherent power over us.

Basking in specific colors can induce feelings and moods that tap into our energy flow and help relieve distress. For instance, red ignites passion and a strong sense of willpower - ideal for individuals who might be struggling with a lack of inspiration or willingness to work as the result of a root chakra blockage.

Some mystics also recommend using tinted glasses to better absorb certain color vibrations in the world around us. Seeing the world through a specific hue can help make it possible to set the mood for your mind. Of course, it also pays to use the colors associated with the chakra you're trying to address.

48th Thing you need to know…

Music

No doubt, there's a way for chakra healing through all of the senses that you might have. And what might surprise you is that each chakra corresponds to specific notes.

There aren't a lot of people who would go as far as measuring the notes of a song or a melody to find out whether it hits the right ones for a specific chakra. But if you're particularly music savvy, then the process might be a treat.

This can get pretty technical though as it includes Solfeggio frequencies and Isochronic Chakra Suite developed through the use of Tibetan singing bowls. Some mystics like to simplify it by leveraging the sound of nature in order to realign a distressed chakra.

Sitting next to flowing, natural bodies of water while you meditate, indulging in the sounds of chirping birds and rustling leaves, or simply basking in the silence of a quite space in your room are just some ways you can use music and sound to heal your chakras.

49th Thing you need to know...

Yoga

Practiced for thousands of years by mystics and Hindu believers, yoga is an excellent, potent method for relieving a chakra blockage. The process of movement, breathing, and maintaining certain postures allows the individual to manipulate the chakras at the subtle plane.

Engaging your body in the correct sequence of movements makes it possible to optimize flow and restore vibrations to their ideal frequencies. There are a variety of types of yoga currently being taught in mainstream studios, but the most effective for chakra relief is Kundalini yoga because of how it combines the physical aspect of an individual to the spiritual facet.

50th Thing you need to know...

Essential Oils

Certain plant extracts exude smells and sensations that are said to cause direct change in the chakras. Because each chakra resonates at a slightly different frequency, using the right kind of oil can help guarantee proper manipulation. Essential oils can be used as scents or as an added feature for chakra massage, depending on how you prefer to leverage their power.

51st Thing you need to know...

Combined Techniques

Using a combination of techniques can help make your journey far more satisfying and rewarding. Knowing how you can blend these methods together can result in more potent outcomes, providing you relief and comfort much sooner than you would have expected.

For instance, during meditation, yoga, or mindfulness, you can incorporate music or sounds. That's why you'll find yoga studios often have indoor fountains that produce soft harmonies of flowing water to help you feel more relaxed and focused as you move. Others also find quiet outdoor spaces where they can hear birds and trees much more conducive to any sort of chakra healing method.

Another way to place yourself in a healing mood more often would be to use scents and essential oils generously throughout your home. Having these aromas flitting about your space for extended periods of time can positively affect your mood and impact your chakras.

Finally, it pays to have your affirmation set ready at all times. Whether it's before a meditation session, right as you're about to go to bed, or just as you wake up in the morning, repeating your positive mantra will help make each and every activity you engage in more meaningful and thus more beneficial for your energy centers.

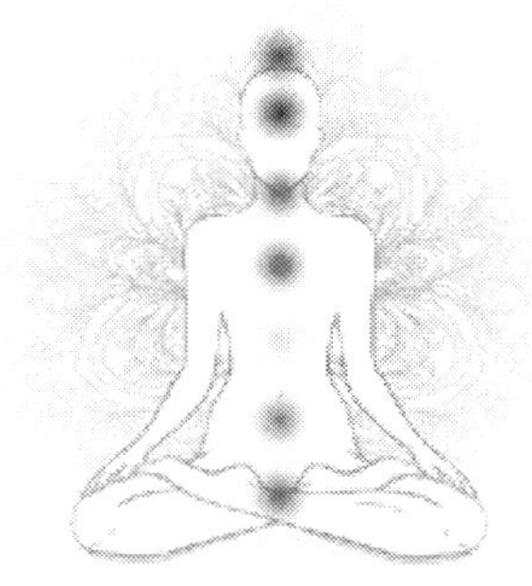

CHAPTER

Seven

Detecting Blocked or Imbalanced Chakras

How exactly do you know if you need to heal something in the first place?

While it's no secret that our chakras become regularly blocked as the result of the many different factors and elements we come into contact with daily, figuring out where a blockage lies isn't something they teach you in school. So, how can you find out whether you need to address a chakra in the first place?

Learning how to diagnose an imbalance or blockage in your energy plexuses improves your insight as to which healing methods you need to implement. Remember - all chakras are different, and each one might respond differently to the strategies you choose.

52nd Thing you need to know...

Develop an Awareness

Who knows yourself better than you? Simply examining your current situation and pinpointing the root of distress can be an effective and accurate means of detecting a blockage or imbalance.

To develop your awareness, simply ask yourself - what area or areas of my life are currently under distress? Does it involve my work? My personal life? My relationships? My family? My mental health? My physical health? My sense of overall satisfaction and well-being?

It's always ideal to localize the issue as precisely as possible in order to develop a specific idea as to which chakra needs to be healed. For instance, a person suffering from dependency problems - either on people or substances - might have a problem with the sacral chakra.

Individuals who are struggling with sinus troubles might have an imbalanced throat chakra.

Take the time to meditate on your situation to get an accurate picture of your current life. Be honest with yourself and be candid about the reality of your circumstances. This will help bring the most pertinent and urgent issues to light.

53rd Thing you need to know...

Examine Your Health

In the same way that the activities you perform in the physical plane have an effect on what you experience in the subtle plane, the status of your chakras can manifest through your physical body. This means that to some extent, it can be assumed that some of the physical ailments and conditions you develop are the result of an insult to the flow of energy through one or more of your chakras.

Have you been feeling under the weather for a while now with no apparent cause? Suffering from disease that has negatively affected your occupational or social functioning? Dealing with constant pangs of pain in different parts of your body? Remember to check which parts of your body certain chakras correspond to - your system might be sending you signals to let you know where the issue lies.

54th Thing you need to know...

Evaluate Your Social Life

Another way that a chakra blockage might make itself known is through your social life. If you're naturally outgoing, friendly, and sociable, and you're noticing a change in the way you usually interact with people around you, it might be an interruption in your chakra.

Of course, not everyone is extroverted by nature. So, what about the people who are more inclined to enjoy time alone? It doesn't have to be such a pronounced change. If you frequently spend time talking to your siblings, a close friend, or if you enjoy scanning through your social media feeds, but start to notice that you're feeling a little more withdrawn than usual, then that could be a sign of an obstruction.

55th Thing you need to know...

Visit a Professional Healer

In our modern world where everything is fueled by consumerist agenda, it's really hard to find legitimate chakra healers. Lots of those you'll find advertised online might actually just be doing it for the monetary gain. This makes it exceptionally challenging to tell whether or not you're chosen healer is actually gifted or not.

Remember though that there are people out there who are naturally talented when it comes to detecting energy blockages. These individuals possess a strong intuition, making them capable of detecting issues with your energy flow more easily than others.

A professional healer can assess you and determine the presence of a blockage, as well as localize the specific problem. They may encourage you to return regularly in order to address the issue and help you achieve relief.

56th Thing you need to know...

Assessing Your Progress

Whether for the short or long term, you probably have a few goals set in place to help guide you towards self-actualization. Maybe you want to improve your work performance, maybe you want to become more sociable, maybe you want to step up your kitchen game. Whatever it might be, these goals help you detect whether or not you're improving or progressing towards the person you want to be.

In many cases, a person might feel stuck and stagnant. Being in the same place with the same level of skill *for months or even years* can feel frustrating and tiring. But there may be a lot more to that feeling of being stuck than you're acknowledging. Try meditating on your life and find out *why* you don't seem to be moving forward. A chakra blockage might be present.

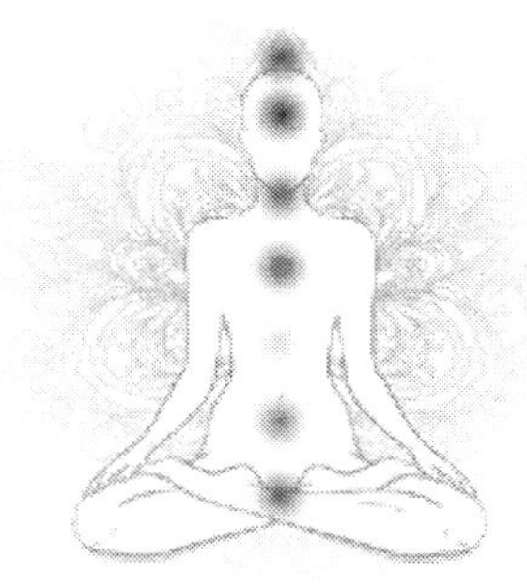

CHAPTER Eight

The Most Common Reasons for Chakra Blockage

Back in the days of ancient Hinduism, balancing energy was a way of life. People would live in rural areas closer to nature and dedicate their lives toward realizing their highest potential. They had very few distractions and were very passionate about their efforts towards becoming their best selves. That's why it wasn't uncommon for older members of their society to reach the higher chakras on the 12 chakra system.

In today's society however, it's rare that you'll find someone who can honestly claim to tap into their soul star chakra or beyond. That's because our world is riddled with distractions that make it hard to truly realize our full spiritual potential.

On top of that, modern life has introduced a variety of factors that make it easier for us to block our own chakras without actually being aware of it. These activities and objects are typical to most of us, which is why we might feel blockages more often than ancient Hindu mystics did.

57th Thing you need to know...

Poor Food Choices

What a lot of people these days don't realize is that *food* is the number one factor contributing to a blocked or imbalanced chakra. Fast food, junk food, and other unhealthy food choices are highly discouraged if you're seeking to balance out a problematic energy plexus.

As a generally accepted notion, *food* inflicts the most potent change on the physical body, which is why many experts and mystics encourage cosmic warriors to be particularly careful of what they put into their system. In the foundations of Kundalini yoga, bad food is the most detrimental to energy health, capable of blotting out power and reducing the flow through your body.

58th Thing you need to know…

Sedentary Lifestyle

The concept of yoga is founded on the idea that your energy can be restored to proper health if you move your body the right way. Movement in the physical plane can generate change in the subtle plane, and yoga aims to encourage proper positioning and breathing techniques in order to change energy flow and develop a more positive balance.

If you're used to sitting around most of the day, it's possible that the flow of energy through your chakras may slow and even stop. Lack of movement is also known to cause blockages as pathways leading to and through chakras might become impinged due to a lack of stimulation.

59th Thing you need to know...

Emotional Distress

Recently broke up with a long-term partner? Had an argument with your mother? Stressing out over something an ex-best friend said about you? You might be feeling particularly distressed, but try not to let it get the best of you.

According to modern experts, this type of insult has the most profound effect on your chakra, and may have you dealing with an imbalance for a while. This is why most mystics and cosmic warriors aim to become more efficient at dealing with emotions and stressful events, because allowing these occurrences to affect you can have a profound impact on your chakras.

60th Thing you need to know...

Physical Injury

Never forget how tantric foundations have changed the way we perceive chakras in modern times. These concepts opened the idea that energy centers have close links to our physical bodies, which is why we can manipulate them with what we do in the physical plane.

In the same light, injury to your body can make it possible to sustain damage to your energy flow. Bodily trauma and disease can send your chakras into distress and discord, which requires immediate physical healing in order to reduce the impact on your energy centers.

61st Thing you need to know...

Chakras Can Be Protected

All around us, there are things that you might call energy "vampires." These factors sap us of our power and make us feel weak. Over time, constant exposure to these objects and activities can lead to severely obstructed chakras that can be particularly difficult to address.

There are a variety of techniques you can put into action in order to avoid these insults. Protecting your chakras from such dangers can help guarantee a seamless flow of energy and a balanced sense of well-being.

62nd Thing you need to know...

Cut Cords

Do you feel particularly connected to a certain energy... in a bad way? Maybe it's your close friend who just ***can't*** stop talking about all the bad things going on in her life, or the next door neighbor who always has something nasty to say about the woman across the street.

Whatever the case, you can sever a tie to help escape the energy link between you and a vampire. Simply find a quiet space in your home, concentrate on the negative energy and try to visualize the ties it has to your aura. With a clear quartz point, move your hand as though cutting the ties while saying something along the lines of, *"I am freeing myself from this negativity. I will only make room for happiness and love in my life."*

63rd Thing you need to know...

Crystal Grids

A crystal grid can take whatever you're feeling and cast it out and away from your space and your life. Choose the right crystals for cleansing, make sure they're the right shape (crystal points are great for directing energy away from you), and endow them with your desired intention. Keep the grid active for as long as you need it to, but make sure to recalibrate it once you reach the 40 day mark.

64th Thing you need to know...

Love Yourself

What an odd and obscure way to free yourself from energy vampires, but it can be highly effective. Often, toxic people in our lives are those who sap most of our positive vibrations with their negative talk and behavior. Unfortunately, humans are naturally inclined to comfort others and lend a listening ear, even if it's detrimental to their own well-being and mental health.

Loving yourself can take a variety of forms, and is almost always guaranteed to help you avoid a toxic person. Set boundaries, learn to say no, acknowledge that *you are not responsible for anyone's happiness*. It doesn't make you any less of a good person if you choose to *put yourself first*.

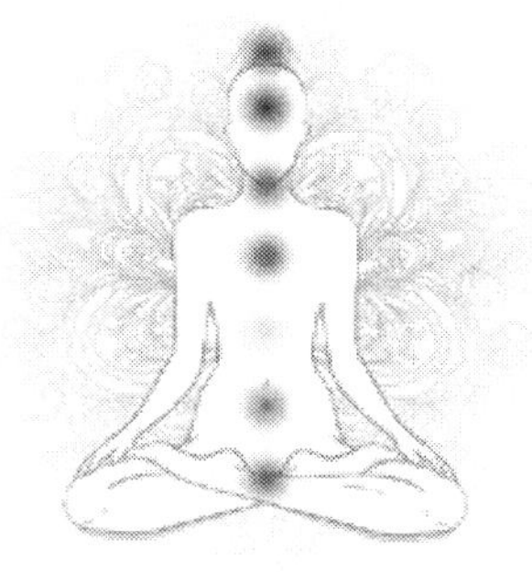

CHAPTER *Nine*

Chakras in Your Home

When they said that chakra healing is a whole life commitment, they mean it extends into every imaginable facet of your life. So aside from your mentality, your physical status, your diet, and your relationships, you can also balance your chakras by making sure your home meets specific standards.

In Asian tradition, the practice of balancing energies in your home is called feng shui, and it closely resembles what experts recommend under the stipulations of modern chakra healing.

65th Thing you need to know...

Cluttered Homes Lead to Blocked Chakras

Imagine yourself walking through your home and seeing boxes upon boxes of your belongings stacked ceiling-high. On the floor are your clothes, shoes, bags, and other personal items, just strewn randomly. Everything is out of place, and a foul smell fills the air making it uncomfortable to stay inside. How do you think you would feel? Stressed out, no doubt.

A cluttered space reflects internal feelings and moods. If you allowed your home to reach such a level of disorganization, it's possible that you might be struggling with internal issues that aren't yet apparent to you. The cluttered aesthetic then increases the feeling of distress, working like a vicious cycle against you.

Making sure you take the time to declutter your home and position your furniture in a way that promotes a free flow of energy can help reduce the distress you feel internally.

66th Thing you need to know...

Root Chakra in Your Home

The root chakra can be represented by your basement. Inhabitants taking shelter in these dark, dingy places can make you feel unsafe and fearful, especially if they're disease riddled vermin like mice or rats. Cleaning it out regularly can make you feel more secure that your home isn't under the attack of potentially dangerous creatures.

67th Thing you need to know...

Sacral Chakra in Your Home

The bedroom is the best representation of the sacral chakra in your home. This is likely where you associate your identity, and is the location where some of the most intimate activities and feelings occur. A cluttered master bedroom can mess with your sense of identity and clarity, and may interfere with your romantic experiences. Making sure it's free of clutter can make it easier for you to find your most important personal belongings, representing clarity of self.

68th Thing you need to know…

Solar Plexus Chakra in Your Home

Your solar plexus chakra can be localized in the bathroom and other personal spaces. These are rooms where you might perform some of the most intimate personal activities, including self-care and rumination. When cluttered or dirty, these rooms can interfere with your feelings of self-confidence and self-worth. Cleaning them out regularly can help guarantee a secure sense of self and potent belief in your own personal power.

69th Thing you need to know…

Heart Chakra in Your Home

The heart chakra exists in the kitchen and dining room where you share some of the most memorable moments in your closest relationships. Here, you share meals and celebrate with relatives and friends, and might have talked most intimately with key people in your life. If the kitchen is cluttered, you might not be able to accommodate people, and thus lose the opportunity to demonstrate love and compassion.

70th Thing you need to know...

Throat Chakra in Your Home

The throat chakra represents communication and interaction with others, which is why it's located in the living room and family room. Here, you're able to share your innermost thoughts and feelings, as well as listen to the ideas of others within the space for healthy debates and discussions. Keeping it well maintained can help facilitate communication and make you feel free to discuss your thoughts with others.

71st Thing you need to know...

Third Eye Chakra in Your Home

The brow/third eye chakra is best represented by the windows in your space. These openings to the outside world are where you can directly perceive what occurs outside of your home - the same way an active third eye allows you to see non-temporal beings and energies. Clean windows allow a much clearer view of the world around you, and give you better insight as to any oncoming weather changes that might require preparation.

72nd Thing you need to know…

Crown Chakra in Your Home

Your attic, rain gutters, and roof are the best representation of your crown chakra at home. Keeping them clean and well-maintained, means you can enjoy the benefits of clarity throughout the rest of your chakra centers. Damaged gutters, leaky roofs, and moldy attics can easily cause destruction on the rest of your home. Hence why it's imperative to ensure that these spaces are always pristine and free from clutter and dirt.

73rd Thing you need to know…

Clean Weekly

If you're feeling tired, weak, uninspired, or stuck, try to examine your home and see how it might reflect your internal feelings. If it's dirty or disorganized, giving it a well-deserved clean may help relieve the way you're feeling. As a part of your whole life change and commitment to optimize your energy flow, make it a point to clean your space at least once a week. This should prevent clutter and filth from accumulating, and may help you experience better energy flow.

74th Thing you need to know...

Consult an Energy Specialist

Even a clean home with minimal clutter can be prone to chakra disruptions. This can happen if items are poorly arranged, or if there are certain energies resonating in specific spaces. Consulting an energy specialist can help give you an insight in to the unique positioning and design issues present in your home.

75th Thing you need to know...

Energy Cleansing

If your space is clean and clutter-free, but you're still sensing some problems with energy flow in specific areas of your home, there might be a negative vibration somewhere in one of the rooms. Lighting up some sage and clearing the space of negative energy can clear up the feelings of heaviness and distress. If the issue persists, consider placing a crystal grid in the room to send out negative vibrations from your space.

76th Thing you need to know...

Incorporate Associations

Remember how specific chakras have unique associations that have particular influence on them? It's always a good idea to incorporate these associations into your space to help in the cleansing of specific chakra blockages you might have detected.

For instance, using green in certain spaces can help resonate with your heart chakra and provide you relief against feelings of loneliness. Using incense throughout your home can improve the relaxation and clarity that you feel when you're in your home.

77th Thing you need to know...

Other Spaces

Aside from your home, it's also important that you make sure the other spaces you frequent are also free from negative energies and factors that could block out your chakras. Your office space, physical store, or your bedroom back at your parents' place should also be subject to regular cleaning and decluttering to guarantee optimal energy movement.

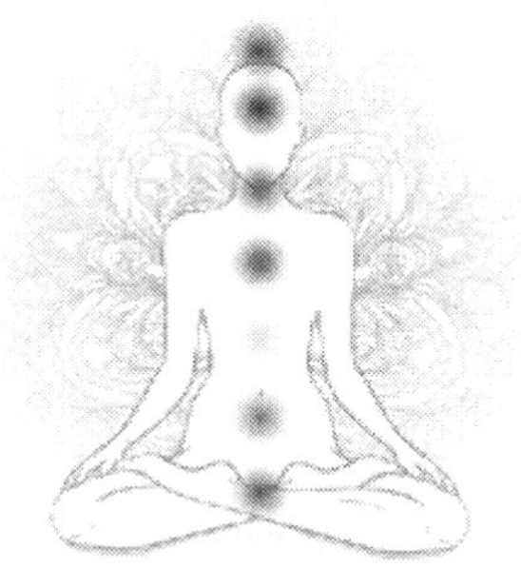

CHAPTER Ten

The Forgotten Chakras

When speaking of chakras, we often focus on just the primary 7 or 12 chakras mentioned by most modern teachers and mystics. But as mentioned earlier in this guide, there are over 88,000 chakras in our bodies, and each one resonates with its own importance and purpose.

While the primary chakras are unique in terms of their significantly more powerful effects on our bodies and souls, there are a few other chakras that are equally noteworthy.

Unfortunately, very few people tap into their power, and thus there are only a handful that know how to use them.

78th Thing you need to know...

Hand Chakras

The hands are some of the most interactive parts of the human body. They allow us to feel the world around us, to provide comfort to a grieving or depressed friend, to express emotion through gestures, and a variety of other functions that many other body parts fail to achieve.

Unlike the 7 (or 12) primary chakras, hand chakras don't have specific names. What we do know about them is that they're present in the wrist, the middle of the palm, and the tips of the 5 fingers.

79th Thing you need to know...

They're Versatile

Each of the 12 primary chakras have unique functions making it easy to detect whether or not they're imbalanced or obstructed.

Unfortunately for hand chakras, that knowledge isn't quite as detailed. All we know is that they do serve a variety of functions.

Firstly, they're used for conveying feelings, emotions, and thoughts. Well balanced hand chakras enable you to communicate freely with individuals around you. They also make you more receptive and sensitive to the feelings and thoughts of others.

Hand chakras also possess the unique quality of allowing you to sense the energy of others. Placing a hand with open chakras on another person can give you a better understanding of their aura, and might even let you perceive specific energy blockages in their subtle body.

Finally, hand chakras can also be used for healing. If you have well balanced energies throughout all of your chakras, and your hand chakras are active and open, you can detect disturbances in other people and transmit positive vibrations to help their healing.

Think of yourself as a unique, living healing crystal, resonating with your own powerful positive vibrations. In fact, this is how a lot of crystal healers help their clients through pranic healing practices.

80th Thing you need to know...

Opening Your Hand Chakras

Not a lot of people focus on opening their hand chakras because they believe that the primary ones are the only ones of importance. But with active hand chakras, you can effectively heal yourself and possibly even become a healing vessel for others.

Sensitive hand chakras can much more easily detect blockages in your other primary chakras. This makes them an essential tool to learn and master if you want to ease the process of clearing out blockages and imbalances.

81st Thing you need to know...

Water Cleansing

It's believed that water can have potent effects on energies, which is why it's often used to cleanse crystals prior to use. Water can neutralize erratic spinning and endow objects with positive energy to make them more useful for healing.

To cleanse your hands, find a flowing body of natural water such as a stream or a river. If there aren't any in your area, a basin of clean water will suffice. Dip your hands into the water and close your eyes. Imagine impurities being washed away, and try to maintain your focus on the feeling of water as it passes over your hands. You can stop the exercise when you start to feel the blockages being lifted away.

82nd Thing you need to know...

Meditation

Specific meditation exercises help bring your hand chakras to your awareness and make it easier to feel them at work. Find a quiet place to sit down and maintain a state of meditation for a few minutes until you feel completely calm and at peace. Once you've achieved clarity, position your hands on your thighs with the palms facing each other.

Focus on how they feel. Try to detect changes in air direction and temperature as you keep your palms open. Now, move them closer together so that they're almost touching. Try to sense each hand using the other without making physical contact, then pull them away again.

During the exercise, you should feel a fuzzy warm feeling in your hands, and you might even be able to sense odd patterns in temperature. Repeating the exercise regularly can help you fine tune your hand chakras for more effective use.

83rd Thing you need to know...

Reiki

One of the practices of Reiki healing has been adapted as an effective method for opening hand chakras. It involves rubbing the palms together until you visualize a ball of light forming between your hands. As you draw the hands apart, imagine the ball remaining in place in the space between your palms. Play with the ball for a while and try to sense its properties. Is it cold? Warm? How does it make your hands feel?

As you end the exercise, bring your hands back together and imagine the ball of light shrinking as you close the gap between your palms. Once your hands are completely together, visualize the light being absorbed back into your body.

84th Thing you need to know...

Artistic Expression

Allowing yourself to freely express art through your hands is another particularly effective method you might want to try. Sculpting, painting, and other modalities that let you create with your hands are some great examples of activities you can perform to open up your hand chakras.

85th Thing you need to know...

Hand Chakras for Healing

Some of the most iconic yoga poses involve the positioning of the open palms so that they're facing outward, away from the body. Why is that so?

Open hand chakras are exceptionally important when it comes to releasing energy from our bodies. When they're active and well-balanced, they serve as entry and exit points for energy, allowing us to transmit positive vibrations and eliminate negative resonance from our bodies.

Once your hand chakras are active, you can use them to eliminate bad vibrations you might sense in your other chakras. For instance, a blocked throat chakra can be addressed by placing the hands over the throat and then speaking an affirmation to relieve the imbalance. Then the hands can take the blockage or stress and cast it out using its active chakras.

Your hand chakras can also be used to heal others. Placing open hand chakras on a friend or relative who's feeling unwell or unhappy can give you an insight as to why they're feeling that way. This can also let you transmit positive vibrations to that person so as to mitigate negativities that might be flowing through their subtle body.

86th Thing you need to know...

Sensing a Healing Aura

If you're not quite confident in your healing capabilities just yet, you might find yourself visiting a psychic healer to help address your chakras. These individuals are said to possess exceptional control and insight regarding their hand chakras, making them highly effective healers.

Before you allow them to work on you though, consider inspecting their aura. Only a person with a clean, free-flowing aura would be able to work away blockages and imbalances in someone else. If they have unhealthy auras, they might actually cause more harm than good.

In this case, you'd be much better off working on yourself.

Which leads us to our final topic.

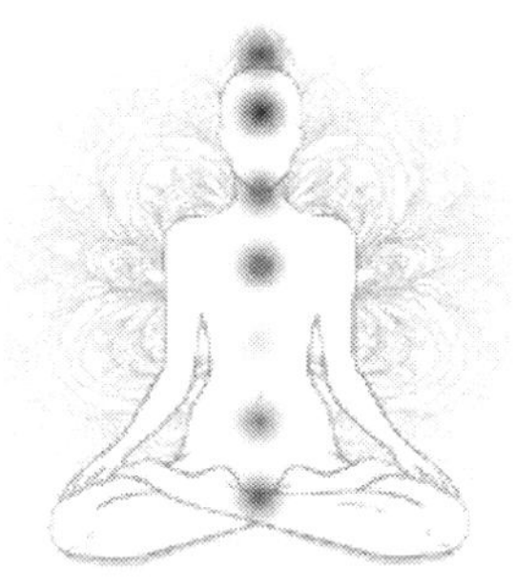

CHAPTER *Eleven*

Chakras and Auras

"You have a beautiful, vibrant aura!" is something you might have heard a psychic healer tell you. Of course, that does sound quite a bit like a compliment, but what is an aura to be exact? And why does it matter to have a clear one?

Unlike chakras, auras don't necessarily affect how you feel, but rather reflect your current state. They shine with colors that represent your feelings, moods, ideas, and your general self-concept at a given time. While your aura might be one color today, it can change tomorrow if you're feeling different about yourself or your situation.

It's important to understand auras because they give you a closer look at the status of your chakras. Disturbances in aura colors betray deeper issues seated in the energy centers of your being.

87th Thing you need to know...

Auras Can Be Perceived

It's hard to tap into *someone else's chakras* because they exist on a deeper plane that's often inaccessible even to the chakras' owner. For instance, you yourself might have difficult accessing your own chakras - how much harder would it be to tap into someone else's?

Conversely, auras can be readily perceived just as long as you have a deeper intuition. It can be highly useful to be able to sense other people's auras because it can give you an idea of the kind of impact they can have on your life.

88th Thing you need to know...

Using Auras to Your Advantage

The capacity to perceive an aura can be particularly important if you're hoping to protect your chakras. Detecting a toxic person by assessing their chakra can help you steer clear of their negativity or mentally prepare yourself for bad vibrations they might send your way.

Similarly, the gift of seeing auras can also be used when faced with a psychic healer. These individuals need to have clear, vibrant auras since they're endowing you with their energies. If they have auras that betray their capacity to provide effective healing, then you might want to seek out a different healer.

89th Thing you need to know...

Training Yourself to See Auras

If you aren't naturally gifted with the talent to see auras, you can try to train yourself to see them. Certain techniques increase your sensitivity to auras and make it possible for you to assess them more accurately. Practicing these techniques - along with your chakra healing practice - can help create a holistic understanding of your spirituality to make you effective at healing not only yourself, but also others around you.

90th Thing you need to know...

Attune to Energies

The first thing you can try to become more aware of the auras of others would be to attune to their energies. The next time you find yourself with a friend or family member, consider sensing the feelings they resonate or encourage. For instance, some friends might make you feel comfortable, light, and happy. Others might make you feel guarded, insecure, and cautious. This gives you an idea as to the kind of energy atmosphere they have around them.

91st Thing you need to know...

Don't Focus Too Hard

One of the pitfalls that most people fall into when trying to learn how to read auras is trying too hard to see them. According to mystics and psychics, you might want to try using your periphery instead of looking at a person head on when you're trying to detect his or her aura. This helps make the colors more perceivable because individuals tend to unconsciously hide their auras when being directly inspected.

92nd Thing you need to know...

Practice on Objects

Everything in the universe resonates with energy, and inanimate objects are no exception. Taking the time to practice on some of the items in and around your space can help you develop your skill and detect more complex auras around you.

The best items to practice with are those with single color auras, such as tumbled crystals. These shine particularly brighter than other objects because of their powerful psychic energies. Place the crystal in a clean, white space and try to focus on it through your periphery. You can also try to look at it directly.

As you observe the crystal, feel free to move it around and play with it in your hands. Maintain your focus on the item, and you will soon start to notice that it resonates with a colorful atmosphere that might be small to start, and then larger and more prominent as you continue.

93rd Thing you need to know...

Aura Qualities

Now that you know how to detect an aura, how can you tell if it's good or bad? There are different qualities to people's auras that give them unique personalities, and allow readers to accurately assess how it translates to a person's current mental, physical, or physical state.

94th Thing you need to know...

Colors and Their Placement

There are lots of different meanings to the colors present in an aura. For instance, black could mean a sign of imminent danger or a previous threat to the health or life of the person being examined. White could represent and advanced connection with specific chakras and energies. Red could point to a passionate, charismatic personality.

The places where the colors are placed also says a lot about the person's aura. A shroud of gray over the heart chakra could mean loneliness and grief, while a bright happy yellow glow around the crown chakra might indicate contentment and joy.

95th Thing you need to know…

Thickness

Some individuals have particularly thick chakras that indicate a strong sense of self and confidence. These people can be infectious and outgoing, allowing them to communicate with others effectively. This is a quality often associated to the auras of politicians or public figures.

Auras that are barely present or that seem very thin and hazy might indicate a problem with confidence and self-esteem. In some cases, it could also indicate a health problem.

96th Thing you need to know…

Chakras and Auras Go Hand In Hand

You can't heal your chakras or the chakras of those around you without first detecting their aura. The importance of knowing the aura is that it showcases the individual's current emotional, physical, and mental status. In knowing this information, you can better understand how to heal their chakras and what specific form of healing they need the most.

Stronger chakras make for stronger auras. The more well-balanced your chakras are, the thicker your aura becomes. This makes it more difficult for negative energies to penetrate your life and cause you distress.

97th Thing you need to know...

Auras Can Be Healed

Just like your chakras, your aura can be healed as well. While it doesn't have a direct impact on your physical body, having a healthy aura can make you more approachable and attractive to people around you. This can help boost your career, increase your chances of finding the right mate, or develop deeper friendships by passively encouraging others to gravitate towards you. Healthy auras can also help transmit positive vibrations, keeping those around you feeling happy and well.

98th Thing you need to know...

Affirmations and Mantras

Before starting the process, you might first have to detect whether your aura needs healing. What colors do you see? How dense is the energy atmosphere around you? And where are the colors positioned? You can do this by sitting next to a mirror and meditating, then focusing on your aura through your peripheral vision. As the colors start to show, try to make a mental note of the aura as you perceive it.

Now, you can develop the appropriate mantra to address the issues you've seen. Something like "I am light and love." can be particularly effective at healing a broken or dull aura. Repeat this to yourself and really feel it in your soul. Try to mean it as deeply as possible with each repetition.

99th Thing you need to know...

Walk in the Rain

Natural sources of water are exceptionally effective at cleansing bad energies and vibrations. Walking in the rain can cleanse your aura and restore your atmosphere to the ideal colors and density. As you walk, try to visualize the rain washing away all the negative vibrations that might be resonating around you. Feel the weight being lifted away, and imagine a clear, bright, vibrant aura take its place.

100th Thing you need to know...

Smudge Yourself with Herbs

Certain herbs can be powerful tools against a blotted out aura. Healing herbs like sage, mint, chamomile, and lavender can help relieve your aura of negative resonance and restore proper balance to your energy atmosphere. To smudge yourself in herbs, simply take a handful of fresh ground leaves or herbal powder and rub them on your body, especially where you detect negative energies in your aura. As you do this, mention your chosen affirmation to completely restore your energies to ideal health.

101st Thing you need to know...

Take a Cleansing Bath

You can also try soaking in an herbal bath to wash away impurities that might have accumulated in your aura as the result of negative forces and experiences. Run a warm bath and infuse your bath water with your chosen herbs. This can be particularly powerful because of the natural cleansing powers of water which has been known to work away negative energies.

The Power to Heal: Conclusion

If there's anything you should take away from these 101 facts, it's that you possess the power to heal. Everything in your life, all of these negative feelings, and every ailment you might be experiencing, whether mental, emotional, or physical - these are all but a drop in the vast ocean that is your life.

Healing is yours for the taking - only if you're willing to make the first step towards understanding and dealing with your energy centers.

Just like an expansive city powered by massive electricity centers, or like lush forests taking power from the sun and streams - your body is an intricate system flowing with energy that fuels your body, your heart, and your spirit. Seeking to optimize the way power flows through these vortexes can help you achieve your best life and become one in mind, body, and soul.

Elizabeth Behnke once said, *"There is deep wisdom within our very flesh, if we can only come to our senses and feel it."* Are you ready to tap into that wisdom?

Cosmic warrior, I hope this comprehensive guide has helped you attain a deeper understanding of your spiritual energy. May this information guide you towards realizing your full potential and becoming the person you've always wanted to be.

Light and love.

Ps. If you enjoyed this book, please leave a review!

Book Preview

CRYSTALS FOR BEGINNERS

The Ultimate Beginners Guide To Understanding and Using Healing Crystals and Stones.

Ella Hughes

Introduction

We're made of star stuff, Carl Sagan once said.

To most of us, his famous words might sound like an unrealistic concept, but they become far more believable when you consider the universe around us and how we came to be.

Created and formed through billions of years of celestial events, the Earth is said to contain the essence of the universe. Carbon, oxygen, and nitrogen are the basic building blocks of life on Earth - and these same elements are believed to have come from the explosive formation of stars some 4.5 billion years ago. But the stars left behind more than these basic ingredients of earth and man.

Underneath our planet's rich soil, tucked away in untouched patches of land, water, and vegetation, collected by those who believe in their unparalleled power - crystals are mysterious objects, shedding light on the bond our planet shares with the stars, and serving as our link to the universe around us.

Crystals have been used for thousands of years through almost every culture and in almost every country. These arcane relics are believed to contain the essence of the stars, allowing them to directly affect the human form. So it's no wonder how the once ancient practice of harnessing the benefits of healing crystals has managed to retain its relevance and purpose in modern times.

From health, to mindfulness, to productivity, and protection - healing crystals have made their own niche in our modern day society. These days, crystals are widely available throughout the market, allowing anyone and everyone to access and attain the benefits they promise.

Are you one of many cosmic warriors hoping to make a place for healing crystals in your life?

In this comprehensive beginner's guide to healing crystals, I will be sharing everything you need to know to get started with the practice. Learn about their mysterious origins and how they were first used in early civilizations. Find out how they work, the science behind their benefits, and how you can use them. And ultimately, discover how the often underestimated power of crystals *can turn your life around and improve every facet of your life.*

This guide shares all the information

essential to starting a healing crystal practice, and provides insight on specific strategies that work best for *each individual person* - allowing you to create a healing crystal practice that truly suits *what you need in your life.*

Ready to unlock your connection with the vast expanse of the universe?

Dive in, cosmic warrior, and let's get started!

CHAPTER One

The Origin of Healing Crystals

Way back when modern medicine was a mystery to most civilized cultures, people used herbal remedies, spiritual practices, and crystals and amulets to heal the sick and to protect against potential disease. These methods were considered sacred and true, until science and medicine were modernized and these original practices were branded obsolete.

However, it's important to understand that for thousands of years, these methods were the only ones that people had - and they worked. So despite the stigma around them, there remain millions who still patronize these practices today.

These days, healing crystals and the powers they contain have become much more mysterious and enigmatic since they're not as commonly used. But that's not how it's always been - especially when you discover just how widespread their benefits once were.

The Earliest Use of Healing Crystals

The earliest traces of the use of healing crystals are dated as far back as 30,000 years ago. Amber from the Baltics was found as far out as Britain, leading researchers to believe that the crystals were considered of such great value that they reached such vast distances. These ancient relics are suspected to have been used as amulets - protecting their owners from disease and illness.

Similarly, researchers have also found crystals buried with the ancient dead throughout various prehistoric communities. Some of the earliest human fossils were found in tombs and graves that were laced with different stones and crystals, which led researchers to conclude that these early humans believed the stones would protect their dead and guide them in the journey through the afterlife.

Some graves - including those found in Switzerland and Belgium - had crystal beads that were fashioned into bracelets and necklaces, which meant that the practice of adorning the body with healing crystals had already been observed as early as the paleolithic era.

While there are still some questions regarding

the reasons why ancient man used crystals, their inherent benefits can't be discounted. And this is proven by their continued popularity throughout the earliest human civilizations.

Healing Crystals in Early Civilizations

Evidence strongly suggests that crystals were used throughout all of the earliest human civilizations currently known. From Sumaria, to Egypt, to ancient Greece, and China, healing crystals had a prominent place in ancient communities as one of the major means towards optimal health and well-being.

The earliest literature describing the use of crystals can be found in ancient Sumarian text where the author describes how the mystical stones were used in magical spells. In Egypt, crystals like lapiz lazuli, turquoise, carnelian, emerald, and quartz were embedded into art, armor, and fashioned into jewelry to protect its wearers.

Pharaohs and other high ranking individuals were buried with a single quartz on their forehead, believed to guide them through the afterlife. Lapiz lazuli, which was strongly associated to one of Egypt's prominent sky goddesses, was usually crushed and worn by women of power since it was believed to enhance awareness and insight. Egyptian women who worked as dancers would place a single ruby on the navel since it was believed to increase sexual appeal.

Ancient Greeks also had quite a few uses for crystals. One of the most noteworthy purposes they found for hematite was to crush it and rub it on the bodies of their warriors prior to battle, since it was said that the stone could protect against injury. Amethyst - which translates literally to 'sober' - was believed to help with ancient hangovers.

Towards the east, healing crystals had a more therapeutic use. Early Chinese communities fashioned small crystal tips onto acupuncture needles which was said to help balance out energies in the body. Crystals were also used in Pranic healing which is practiced even in modern times - some 5,000 years later.

A Sustained Prominence in the Years AD

In the Renaissance, mystic healers continued to harness the energy of crystals and used them for a variety of health conditions. Some literature described how healing crystals were used in medicine and most of the authors including Binghen, Saxo, and Mandeville often cited that the benefits of crystals became much more potent when used alongside herbal healing practices.

During this time, crystals were seen as endowed with 'virtues' which could be corrupted. Some mystics believed that Adam's original sin caused some gemstones to lose their virtue. Others thought that a crystal's inherent virtue could be lost if used improperly or if handled by a sinner.

In this light, crystals in the Renaissance were used with utmost caution and care. Before their powers were harnessed, stones were cleansed, consecrated, and sanctified - a practice reflected in today's process of cleansing and programming crystals prior to use.

Some crystals in the period of the Renaissance were particularly valuable. One such relic was a gem in the possession of Henry III which was allegedly stolen by his chief jesticular. The gem was said to have been given to the King of Wales - Henry's enemy. This angered Henry, and the jesticular was branded a criminal since the gem he had stolen was considered most powerful, capable of making its wearer invincible.

The Renaissance was a colorful period of learning. So as people grew more and more intelligent in their sciences and arts, many wanted to learn how exactly crystals had an effect on the human form. It was during the Age of Enlightenment that Thomas Nicols started the movement towards more scientific methods of medicine and healing with his *Faithful Lapidary*.

In his iconic text, Nicols described that gems, as inanimate objects, couldn't possess the powers and effects that people originally believed they had. And that's when the interest in crystal healing began to decline.

The Rebirth of Gemstone Use

It took around a century and a half before gemstones would once again find their place as a mainstream form of healing and wellness. In the 80s and 90s, western authors made the use of healing crystals prominent once more, reigniting the public's interest in their mystical power and effects.

Of course these days, the use of crystals is widely considered a pseudoscience. However, their prominence throughout thousands of years of civilization makes it difficult to debunk their inherent, arcane effects. Plus, with the advancement of science and research, it has become possible to back the benefits of crystals with real, *tangible evidence* - a factor that was unfortunately, unavailable in Nicols' time.

If you'd like to keep reading, please click here.

Other books you might enjoy!

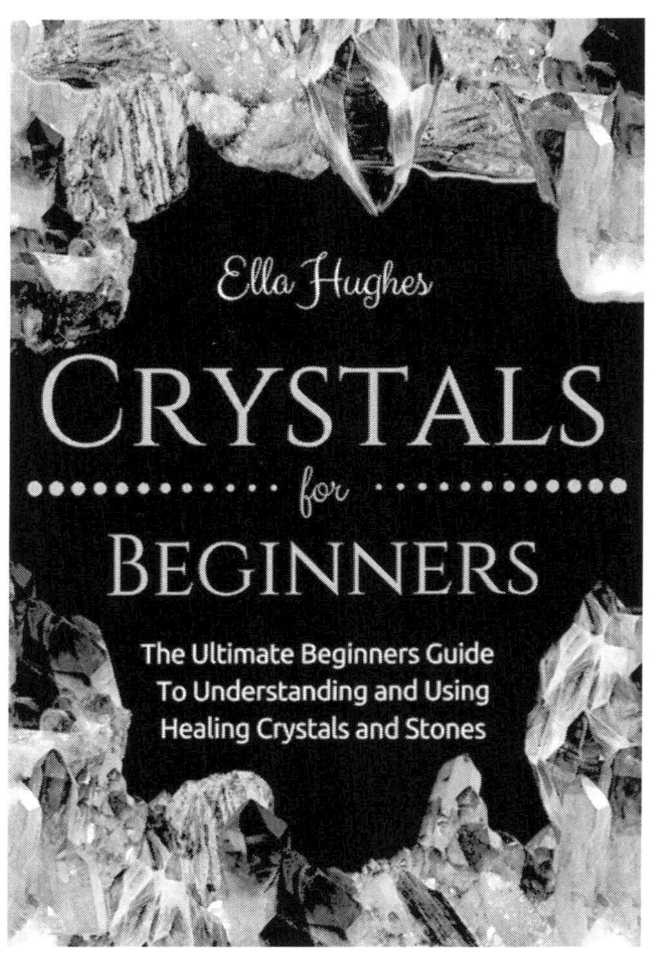

Crystals for Beginners: The Ultimate Beginners Guide To Understanding and Using Healing Crystals and Stones.

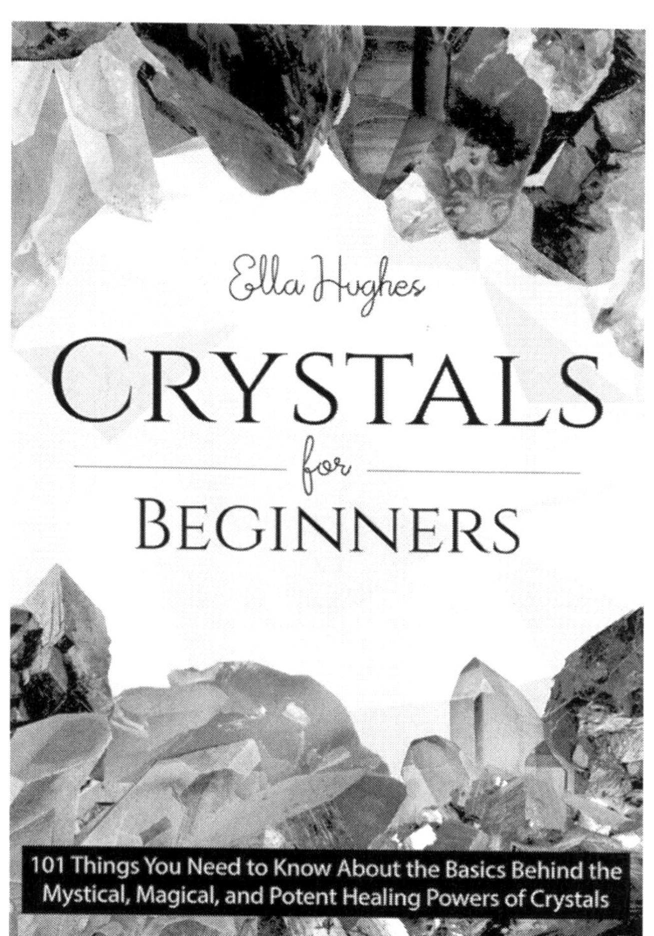

Crystals for Beginners: 101 Things You Need to Know About the Basics Behind the Mystical, Magical, and Potent Healing Powers of Crystals

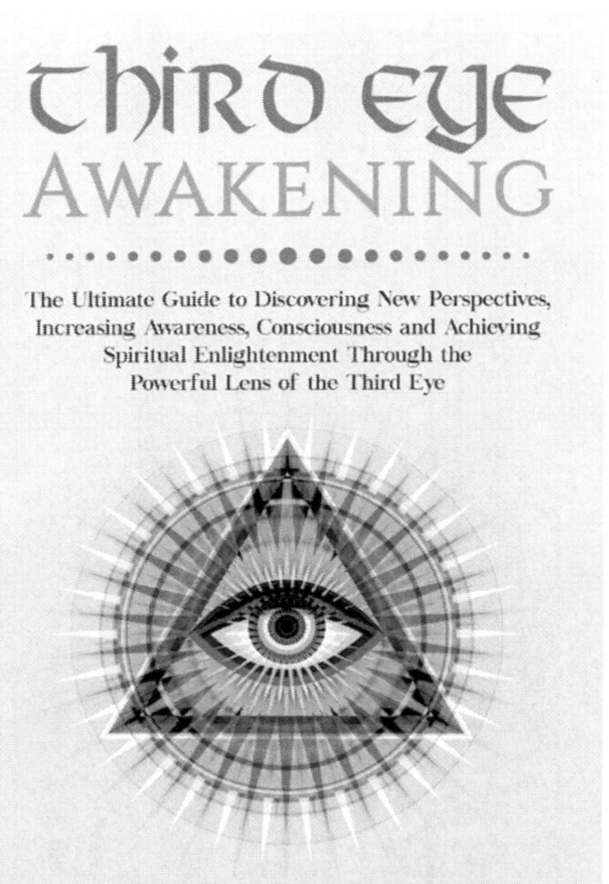

Third Eye Awakening: The Ultimate Guide to Discovering New Perspectives, Increasing Awareness, Consciousness and Achieving Spiritual Enlightenment Through the Powerful Lens of the Third Eye

Printed in Great Britain
by Amazon